Mediterranean Sweet Moments

50 Easy & Delicious Mediterranean Recipes for Your Breakfast & Sweet Moments

Jenna Violet

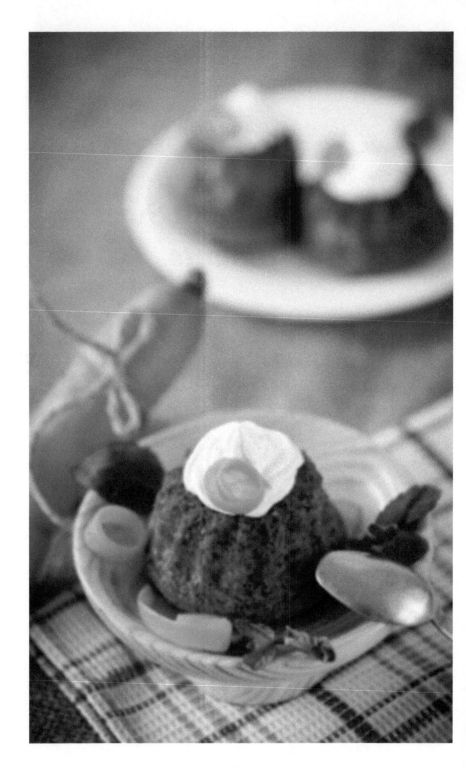

Table of Contents

Clumpy granola with stewed rhubarb

Ingredients

- 2 tablespoons of maple syrup
- ½ cup of almonds, chopped
- ½ cup of puffed brown rice
- ½ cup of chickpea flour
- 1 vanilla bean pod, scraped
- ¼ cup of pepitas
- 2 rhubarb stalks, trimmed and cut pieces
- ¼ cup of sunflower seeds
- 1 teaspoon of ground cinnamon
- 2 cups of old-fashioned oats
- 2 teaspoons of lemon juice
- 1 teaspoon of ground ginger
- ½ teaspoon of ground nutmeg
- ½ teaspoon of sea salt
- Scant ½ cup of maple syrup
- Scant ½ cup of melted coconut oil

Directions

- Start by preheating your oven to 300°F, then line a large baking sheet with parchment paper.
- Next, in a large mixing bowl, combine the oats together with the almonds, puffed rice, sunflower seeds, chickpea flour, pumpkin seeds, nutmeg, cinnamon, ginger, and salt. Mix to blend.
- In another smaller bowl, whisk together the maple syrup and coconut oil until combined.
- Pour the wet mixture into the dry, and mix well.
- Move the granola to the prepared baking sheet and use the back of a big spoon to spread it out into an even layer.
- Let bake for about 40 minutes, rotating the pan halfway through, until golden and fragrant.
- Allow the pan to cool completely to keep the clumps intact.

- Gently break up the granola into clumps and store in an airtight container at room temperature for up to 2 weeks or in a freezer.
- Then, heat a medium saucepan over medium-low heat.
- Add the rhubarb together with the maple syrup, lemon juice, and vanilla bean, and stir to mix.
- Cover let cook for 10 minutes, stirring occasionally, until the mixture is bubbling and the rhubarb is tender. Keep aside for later.
- Divide the yogurt between 4 bowls
- Then, add ½ cup granola to each bowl and then divide the stewed rhubarb into the bowls.
- Serve and enjoy.

Blueberry baked oatmeal

Ingredients

- 2 teaspoons of raw sugar
- 2 teaspoons of ground cinnamon
- 12 ounces of fresh or frozen blueberries
- 1 teaspoon baking powder
- Vanilla yogurt
- ¾ teaspoon of fine-grain sea salt
- ¼ teaspoon of ground nutmeg
- ⅔ cup of roughly chopped pecans
- 1 ¾ cups of milk of choice
- ⅓ cup of maple syrup or honey
- 2 large eggs or flax eggs
- 2 cups of old-fashioned oats
- 3 tablespoons of melted unsalted butter
- 2 teaspoons of vanilla extract

Directions

- Expressly, preheat your oven ready to 375°F.
- Then, oil a square baking dish .

- Pour the nuts onto a rimmed baking sheet when the oven has finished preheating, let toast for 5 minutes, until fragrant.
- In a medium mixing bowl, combine the oats together with the, toasted nuts, cinnamon, baking powder, salt and nutmeg. Mix to combine.
- In another separate smaller mixing bowl, combine the milk, maple syrup, egg, half of the butter, and vanilla. Mix until blended.
- Reserve about ½ cup of the berries for topping the baked oatmeal, then arrange the remaining berries evenly over the bottom of the baking dish
- Cover the fruit with the dry oat mixture, then drizzle the wet ingredients over the oats.
- Wiggle the baking dish to make sure the milk moves down through the oats, then gently pat down any dry oats resting on top.
- Scatter the remaining berries across the top.
- Sprinkle some raw sugar on top for extra sweetness and crunch.

- Let bake for 45 minutes, until the top is nice and golden.
- Remove your baked oatmeal from the oven.
- Allow it to cool for briefly for few minutes.
- Then, drizzle with the remaining melted butter on the top.
- Serve and enjoy.
- Any left overs can be kept in the fridge for up to 5 days.

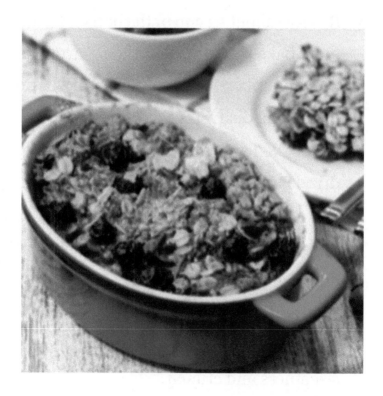

Healthy carrot muffins

Ingredients

- ½ cup of maple syrup or honey
- 1 teaspoon of ground cinnamon
- ½ teaspoon of salt
- 1 tablespoon of turbinado sugar
- ⅓ cup of melted coconut oil
- ½ teaspoon of ground ginger
- 1 teaspoon of vanilla extract
- ¼ teaspoon of ground nutmeg
- 1 ¾ cups of white whole wheat flour
- 1 cup of plain Greek yogurt
- 2 eggs, preferably at room temperature
- 1 ½ teaspoons of baking powder
- ½ teaspoon of baking soda
- 2 cups of peeled and grated carrots
- ½ cup of roughly chopped walnuts
- ½ cup of raisins tossed in 1 teaspoon flour

Directions

- Preheat oven to 425°F.

- Grease all the 12 cups on the muffin tin with butter.
- In a large mixing bowl, combine the flour together with the baking powder, cinnamon, baking soda, salt, ginger and nutmeg. Blend with a whisk.
- In a separate, small bowl, toss the raisins with 1 teaspoon flour to avoid sticking together.
- Add the grated carrots together with the chopped walnuts and floured raisins to the other ingredients and stir to combine.
- In another separated medium sized mixing bowl, combine the oil and maple syrup, let whisk together.
- Add the eggs and beat well, then add the yogurt together with vanilla, mix well.
- Mix the wet ingredients together with the dry ones then mix with a big spoon, to combine.
- Divide the batter evenly between the 12 muffin cups.
- Sprinkle the tops of the muffins with turbinado sugar.

- Let bake for 16 minutes, until the muffins are golden on top and a toothpick inserted into a muffin comes out clean.
- Place the muffin tin on a cooling rack to cool.
- Serve and enjoy.
- The muffins when frozen, can last for up to 3 months.

Cranberry orange granola bars

Ingredients

- ¾ teaspoon of salt
- 1 cup of pecan pieces
- 1 ½ teaspoons of vanilla extract
- ⅔ cup of dried cranberries
- ½ cup of honey
- 1 ¾ cups of quick-cooking oats
- 1 teaspoon of orange zest, preferably organic
- 1 cup of creamy unsalted almond butter or peanut butter, packed
- ½ teaspoon of ground cinnamon
- ⅓ cup of pepitas

Directions

- Firstly, line a square baker with two strips of crisscrossed parchment paper, cut to fit neatly against the base and up the sides.
- In a medium skillet over medium heat, toast the pecans and pepitas, stirring often, until they are fragrant in 5 minutes.

- Move the toasted pecans and pepitas to a food processor.
- Then, add the cranberries and then run the machine for about 10 seconds, until the nuts and cranberries are all broken up.
- In a mixing bowl, combine the contents of the food processor together with the oats, orange zest, cinnamon and salt. Mix to combine.
- In another separate smaller mixing bowl, mix together the almond butter, honey and vanilla extract until well blended.
- Mix the liquid ingredients together with the dry ingredients.
- Use a big spoon to mix them together until the two are evenly combined and no dry oats remain.
- Shift the mixture to the prepared square baker.
- By the Use of a spoon, arrange the mixture fairly evenly in the baker.
- Then, use the bottom of a flat, round surface covered in a small piece of parchment paper,

to pack the mixture down as firmly and evenly as possible.

- Cover the baker and refrigerate for 2 hours or overnight for the best outcome.
- To slice, lift the bars out of the baker by grabbing both pieces of parchment paper on opposite corners.
- With a sharp knife, slice the bars into strips, then slice them in half through the middle.
- Serve and enjoy.
- Any left overs can be kept in the fridge for days.

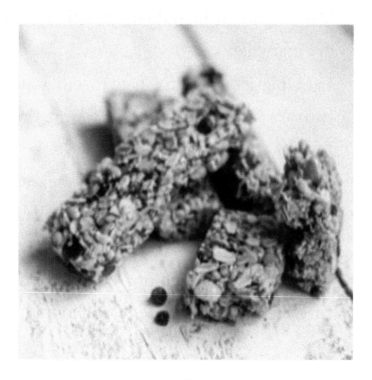

Butternut squash frittata with fried sage

Ingredients

- Freshly ground black pepper
- 16 fresh sage leaves
- 2 cloves garlic
- ¾ cup of freshly grated Parmesan
- 3 tablespoons of extra-virgin olive oil
- 8 eggs
- ¾ pound of butternut squash
- ½ cup of milk
- ¾ cup of chopped yellow onion
- ¾ teaspoon of sea salt, divided

Directions

- Preheat the oven ready to 425°F.
- In a large bowl, whisk together the eggs together with the milk, garlic, teaspoon salt, and several twists of freshly ground black pepper and half of the cheese.
- In a well-seasoned cast iron skillet, warm 1 tablespoon olive oil over medium heat.
- Add the chopped onion, stir to coat.

- Let cook for a few minutes, until the onions are starting to turn translucent.
- Add the squash and ½ teaspoon salt and stir to mix.
- Cover the pan and reduce heat, let cook for 8 minutes as you stir occasionally.
- Uncover the pan, raise the heat back to medium continue to cook until the excess moisture has evaporated in about 6 or 10 minutes.
- Lower the heat.
- Arrange the butternut in an even layer in the bottom of the skillet.
- Then, whisk the egg mixture one last time and pour it into the pan.
- Sprinkle the frittata with the remaining cheese.
- Put the pan in the oven and bake until you can shake the pan and you can the middle is just barely set in 17 minutes.
- Then, heat oil in a large skillet over medium heat.

- Once the oil is shimmering, add the sage and toss to coat.
- Let the sage get crispy then transferring it to a plate covered with a paper towel.
- Sprinkle the fried sage lightly with sea salt and set it aside.
- Sprinkle fried sage on top and let the frittata rest a few minutes, then slice into 8 smaller wedges.
- Serve and enjoy.

Mango panna cotta

Though a perfect Mediterranean Sea diet, mango panna cotta an Italian desert wonderful picnics, parties and dinners. It can be prepared ahead of time.

Ingredients

- A knob of butter
- ½ cup of whole milk
- ½ teaspoon of vanilla essence
- 1 cup of heavy cream the whole package
- 1 packet gelatin
- ½ lemon, juice only
- 2 cups of frozen mango chunks, thawed
- ⅓ cup of granulated sugar
- 2 tablespoons of granulated sugar

Directions

- Pour heavy cream together with the milk and sugar into a small sauce pan.
- Stir to dissolve the sugar on over low heat, the cream should be hot.
- Turn off the heat and stir vanilla essence. Make sure not to boil at this stage.

- The bloom should be gelatin as per the package Directions.
- Add the bloomed gelatin to the cooled cream mixture. Do not forget to mix to dissolve.
- Pour the mixture into small glasses, place to refrigerate to set the panna cotta for 2 hours.
- Process the thawed mango pieces together with the lemon juice and sugar in a blender until smooth.
- Taste and adjust accordingly.
- Simmer in a small saucepan over low heat.
- Stir in butter to get a much creamier texture.
- Allow the mixture to cool.
- Pour over the panna cotta.
- Serve and enjoy.

Candied oranges dipped in chocolate

This recipe is for a sweet tasty treat for a perfect holiday to enjoy Mediterranean Sea diet. The chocolates can be substituted with cupcakes if you like.

Ingredients

- 3.5 ounces of Dark Chocolate
- 1 Large Orange, organic
- Coarse Salt
- 1 cup of Granulated Sugar
- 1 cup of Water

Directions

- Cut the oranges into thin slices.
- Heat water and sugar in a large pot until the sugar has dissolved.
- Add the orange slices in a manner that they are spread around without covering each other totally.
- Let simmer for 40 minutes on a low heat. Turn occasionally.
- Transfer slices onto a wire rack when ready, let them cool completely.

- It is fine to cool on a fridge to speed up the cooling process.
- Melt the chocolate over a pot of simmering water.
- Dip half of each slice in chocolate.
- Place the dipped one's onto a tray lined with a sheet of aluminum foil.
- Sprinkle with salt.
- Shift all of them into the fridge.
- Serve an enjoy.

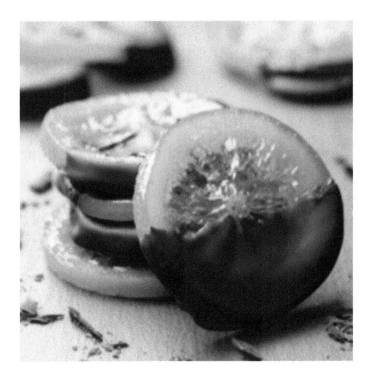

Walnut crescent cookies

If you want taste and know divine taste covered in a powdered sugar, look no further, walnut crescent cookies can give you that same exact taste.

Ingredients

- 2 tablespoons of vanilla sugar
- 11/4 cup of all-purpose flour
- ½ cup of powdered sugar
- 1 stick unsalted butter
- ⅔ cup of ground walnuts
- 4 tablespoons of powdered sugar
- 1 teaspoon of vanilla essence

Directions

- In a large mixing bowl, begin by combining sifted powdered sugar, sifted flour, and ground walnuts.
- Next, add vanilla essence and mix thoroughly.
- Then, grate chilled butter.
- Add to the bowl.

- Combine all the ingredients using your bare hands until dough is formed in 3 minutes or so.
- Place into a Ziploc bag allow it to chill for 30 minutes in the fridge.
- As it refrigerates, get a small bowl and place extra powdered sugar with vanilla sugar in it and keep aside.
- Take a piece of the dough and roll into a ball then into a sausage.
- Shape the sausage into a crescent.
- Place onto a baking tray with baking parchment.
- For the remaining dough, repeat this step.
- Bake in a ready heated oven at 400°F for 8 minutes or so.
- Allow it to cool down completely on the tray when already fried.
- Transfer to a plat and dip with powdered sugar to coat.
- Serve and enjoy.

Caramel apple dip

The caramel apple dip is a perfect and excellent choice for family gatherings with only 3 ingredients, it is a quickie in only 2 minutes with absolutely no cooking and frying needed.

Ingredients

- Caramels
- ½ cup of Dulce de leche
- 2 – 3 apples, cut into small pieces
- ½ cup of cream cheese

Directions

- In a bowl, mix the cream cheese together with the Dulce de leech until smooth.
- Cut the apples into quarters after rinsing.
- Remove the hard parts.
- Further cut every quarter into 6 slices
- Serve and enjoy.

Easy lemon cupcakes

Lemon is a nutritious fruit fantastic for a Mediterranean Sea diet. The lemon gives this recipe a flavorful taste super moist topped with vanilla mascarpone cream cheese frosting.

Ingredients

- ½ cup of granulated sugar
- 3/4 cup of all-purpose flour
- 2 eggs, at room temperature
- 2 teaspoon of baking powder
- 1/4 teaspoon of vanilla essence
- 3 small lemons, juice only
- A pinch of salt
- ½ cup of powdered sugar
- 1 tablespoon of lemon juice
- 1 stick unsalted butter , softened
- 9 ounces of mascarpone cheese
- ½ cup of cream cheese

Directions

- Firstly, begin by preheating your oven to 360°F.

- Juice all the lemons without the seeds, keep for later.
- In a mixing dish, beat the butter together with sugar until creamy in 3 minutes.
- Add the eggs and mix well.
- Combine the flour together with the baking powder and salt.
- Add this to the cupcake batter and mix until smooth.
- Pour in the lemon juice and mix thoroughly for the last time.
- Place the paper cases in a muffin tray.
- Using a pipe, pipe the batter into paper cases.
- Let bake for 15 minutes.
- If you the inserted skewer comes out clean, it is an indication that the cupcakes are ready.
- Remove from the oven.
- Pour in the balance of the lemon juice over each cupcake (2 spoons per cake).
- Allow it to cool down completely.
- Shift all the ingredients into a mixing bowl.

- Combine them using an electric mixer until smooth.
- Serve and enjoy.

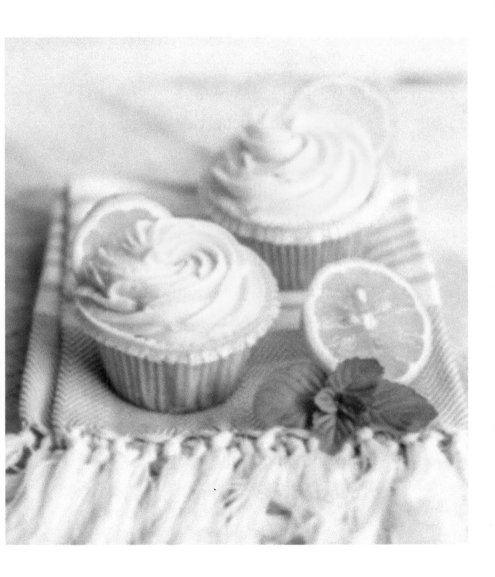

Lemon blueberry poke cake from scratch

This is a typical moist sponge soft recipe featuring blueberry sauce and creamy ricotta with a hint of lemon to give it the attractive flavor for a Mediterranean Sea diet.

Ingredients

- ½ cup of powdered sugar
- 1½ teaspoon of baking powder
- 1 cup of fresh blueberries
- ½ lemon, juice only
- 1/4 cup of sunflower oil
- 1/4 cup of water
- 1 cup of all-purpose flour
- 3 medium eggs, yolks and whites separated
- ½ cup of granulated sugar
- 2 cups of frozen blueberries
- Lemon zest
- 3/4 cup of granulated sugar
- ½ lemon, juice only
- 8 ounce of mascarpone
- 1/4 cup water
- 8 ounce of ricotta

Directions

- Start by beating the egg whites until soft peaks forms, keep for later.
- In another separate mixing dish, whisk the egg yolks together with sugar until creamy.
- Sift in flour mixed with baking powder. Mix properly.
- Add oil together with water, continue to mix with an electric mixer until smooth.
- Fold in the egg whites and pour the batter in a rectangular baking dish.
- Begin baking for 15 minutes at 375°F.
- Allow it to cool down.
- Pierce in holes when completely cooled.
- As the cake is in the oven, heat up the blueberries together with the water, sugar, and lemon juice in a sauce pan.
- Over low heat simmer for 7 minutes.
- Turn off heat, keep aside.
- In another separate bowl, combine ricotta together with the freshly squeezed lemon juice, mascarpone, and sugar.

- Place in the electric mixer mix until well combined.
- Pour the blueberries and their juice over the cake sponge.
- Then, spread the ricotta layer over.
- Refrigerate to chill.
- Serve and enjoy with blueberries and or grated lemon zest if you like.

Chocolate mango cheesecake parfait

This is an excellent choice for passing through the summer season. It combines Oreo cookies with fresh mangoes, mango cheesecake and chocolate for a tastier breakfast for a Mediterranean diet.

Ingredients

- 3 tablespoons of lemon juice
- 1 fresh mango
- 12 ounces of cream cheese
- 1 packet of Oreo cookies
- ½ cup of whipping cream
- 2 tablespoons of unsweetened cocoa powder
- ½ cup of powdered sugar

Instruction

- Begin by cutting the mango, scoop the flesh from one half out.
- Puree in a food processor, keep aside.
- The remaining half should be cut into slices.
- Whip the cream until soft peaks form in a small mixing dish.

- Add the cream cheese together with the powdered sugar and mix to combined.
- Divide this mixture equally between 2 dishes.
- Add pureed mango and lemon juice in one.
- Fill the next one with cocoa powder.
- Mix both until well combined.
- You can start with a whole Oreo cookie.
- Then a mango cheesecake layer, fresh mango slices.
- Then, lastly, place the chocolate cheesecake layer.
- Repeat this until everything is finished.
- Garnish with some Oreo crumb.
- Refrigerate for 1 hour to chill.
- Serve and enjoy.

Mango tiramisu

This a Mediterranean delicious fruity version of the Italian classic desert. It features mango sauce, mascarpone mixture and layers of ladyfingers finished with cocoa or mango slices in 30 minutes.

Ingredients

- 12 ounce of mascarpone cheese
- 9 ounce of sour cream
- 1 cup of hot water
- 1/4 cup of water
- 2 teaspoons of instant coffee
- 4 tablespoons of vanilla sugar
- 2 cups of fresh mango pieces
- 5 tablespoons of granulated sugar
- ½ medium lemon, juice only
- 7 ounce of ladyfingers

Directions

- Mix your coffee with hot water in a jug. Allow it to cool down in totality.
- As the coffee cooling, put diced mango in a sauce pan

- Add sugar and water.
- Over low heat, simmer the mixture for 4 minutes.
- Turn off the heat.
- Shift the content into a bowl, add juice from half a lemon
- Using a fork, mash the mango. Stir and let it cool down.
- Combine the mascarpone together with the sour cream and vanilla sugar in a dish.
- Mix this until smooth, preferably using an electric mixer.
- Get a loaf tin and line it with aluminum foil.
- Pour the coffee into a shallow plate.
- Immediately dip each ladyfinger in it.
- Cover the whole bottom of the tin with ladyfingers.
- Spread over about a third of the mascarpone mixture.
- Top with chilled mango sauce.
- Repeat until everything is done.

- Refrigerate the tiramisu in a fridge for at 3 hours.
- Dust the top with cocoa powder.

Serve and enjoy with mango slices garnished on top.

Raspberry mint ice pops

Mint is one element in this recipe that gives it a refreshing taste and keeping you hooked onto it. The raspberry flavor can be felt through the entire raspberry.

Ingredients

- 1½ cup of Fresh Raspberries
- 1 Wedge of Lemon
- ⅓ cup of Honey
- 10 Mint Leaves
- 1 cup of Water

Directions

- In a small sauce pan, combine the honey, water, together with 5 mint leaves.
- Heat this up without boiling until the honey is melted. Keep for later.
- Then, puree the raspberries including the remaining mint leaves in a food processor.
- Sieve the mixture to remove any seeds in it.
- Make sure to remove any mint leaves from honey water at this stage.
- Add in the pureed raspberries.

- Squeeze in the lemon mix thoroughly.
- Then pour it into popsicle molds.
- Freeze for at least 8 hours, otherwise 12 hours is best.
- Serve and enjoy.

Honey lemony ricotta breakfast toast with figs and pistachios

Ingredients

- ¼ cup of low fat ricotta
- 2 tablespoons of pistachio pieces
- 1 teaspoon of lemon zest
- ½ fresh of lemon, juiced
- ½ tablespoon of honey
- 2 slices whole grain
- 4 figs, sliced

Directions

- Toast bread in toaster.
- Whip together ricotta, lemon juice and honey until smooth and creamy.
- Spread ricotta moisture evenly over each piece of toast.
- Top with sliced figs.
- Sprinkle each piece with pistachio pieces and lemon zest.
- Serve and enjoy.

Baked eggs with avocado and feta

Ingredients

- salt and fresh-ground black
- Olive oil
- 4 eggs
- 1 avocado
- 2 tablespoons of crumbled feta cheese

Directions

- Break eggs into individual ramekins.
- Let eggs and avocado come to room temperature for 15 minutes.
- Set the oven to 400F.
- Put the gratin dishes on a baking sheet and heat them in the oven for 10 minutes.
- Peel the avocado and cut each half into 6 slices.
- Remove gratin dishes from the oven and spray with olive oil.
- Arrange the sliced avocados in each dish and tip two eggs into each dish.
- Sprinkle with crumbled feta.

- Season to taste with salt and fresh-ground black pepper.
- Let bake for 12 until the whites are set.
- Serve and enjoy hot.

Avocado Caprese wrap

Ingredients

- balsamic vinegar
- 2 whole wheat tortillas
- 1 ball fresh mozzarella cheese sliced
- kosher salt and freshly ground black pepper
- olive oil
- ½ cup of fresh arugula leaves
- 1 tomato sliced
- 1 avocado pitted and sliced
- basil leaves

Directions

- Layer slices of tomato together with the mozzarella cheese and avocado on the tortilla.
- Add a few torn pieces of basil leaves.
- Drizzle with olive oil and balsamic vinegar.
- Season with kosher salt and pepper,
- Fold the tortilla in thirds.
- Serve and enjoy.

Caprese avocado toast

Directions

- Flaked sea salt
- 1 slice whole-wheat toast
- Basil leaves
- 2 teaspoons of flaxseed oil
- 1 small tomato
- ½ avocado, peeled and sliced
- 1/3 cup of low-fat cottage cheese

Directions

- Begin by toasting your bread
- Drizzle with flaxseed oil.
- Layer with the avocado, cottage cheese and tomato.
- Garnish with basil leaves and flaked sea salt.
- Serve and enjoy.

Saucy Greek baked shrimp

Ingredients

- ½ teaspoon of ground cinnamon
- ½ teaspoon of ground allspice
- 1 pound large peeled and deveined shrimp
- ½ teaspoon of red pepper flakes
- ¼ teaspoon of kosher salt
- 2 tablespoons of chopped fresh dill
- 3 tablespoons of olive oil
- ½ cup of crumbled feta cheese
- 3 garlic cloves pressed or minced
- 1 15- ounce can of crushed tomatoes
- 1 medium onion chopped

Directions

- Preheat your oven ready to 375°F.
- Pat dry the shrimp and place in a bowl.
- Season with the red pepper flakes and kosher salt, keep aside.
- Drizzle the olive oil in a heavy skillet and heat over medium heat.

- Add the onion and garlic and cook until softened in 5 minutes.
- Stir in the spices let cook for 30 seconds.
- Add the tomatoes and simmer, uncovered, for about 20 minutes, stirring occasionally.
- Remove from the heat.
- Put shrimp into the tomato sauce and crumble the feta cheese over the top.
- Let bake for 18 minutes until cooked through.
- Sprinkle with the dill.
- Serve and enjoy with crusty bread.

Mango yogurt popsicles

This is per harps the most refreshing Mediterranean Sea diet healthiest mango drink with simple and easy to make ingredients. It is also perfect for the summer.

Ingredients

- 1 stick of unsalted butter
- 5 ounces of milk chocolate
- 1 cup of Greek yogurt
- 1 wedge lemon
- 1/4 cup of granulated sugar
- 2½ cups of frozen mango pieces, slightly thawed

Directions

- Combine the yogurt together with lemon juice, sugar, and mango pieces in a food processor.
- Process until smooth.
- Pour the mixture in a popsicle mold with inserted sticks.
- Place in the freezer overnight.
- Remove the popsicles, allow then to heat to room temperature for a few minutes.

- Take out of the molds.
- Place a sheet of parchment paper in the freezer and place the popsicles onto it.
- Cut the chocolate into tiny pieces, place all of them a dish.
- Add diced butter and melt over a double boiler.
- Pour this melted chocolate into mug that is preferably heat proof for dipping each popsicle.
- As you take out, allow the excess chocolate to gently drip back.
- Make sure to repeat this very step with all the reaming popsicles.
- Place the ready ones back in the freezer.
- Remove, let settle to a bit.
- Serve and enjoy.

Banana bread

Banana is a fruit of the heart blessed with abundant fiber. Above and beyond, it is moist, soft and sweet. It is best with honey or butter depending on how you like it.

Ingredients

- A few drops of vanilla essence
- ½ cup of granulated sugar
- 1 large egg
- 1½ cup of all-purpose flour
- 1 teaspoon of baking soda
- 3 large ripe bananas
- ⅓ cup of unsalted butter
- 1 teaspoon of ground cinnamon

Directions

- Begin by preparing the bananas, cut them into small pieces.
- Put them in a medium sized dish, then mash them with a fork.
- Add in large egg, beaten with a fork. Mix properly.

- Add baking soda along with the melted butter, caster sugar, vanilla essence, flour. Make sure you mix well.
- Pour the batter into a loaf tin lined with baking paper.
- Place in a preheated oven and bake for 1 hour at 355°F.
- Serve and enjoy.

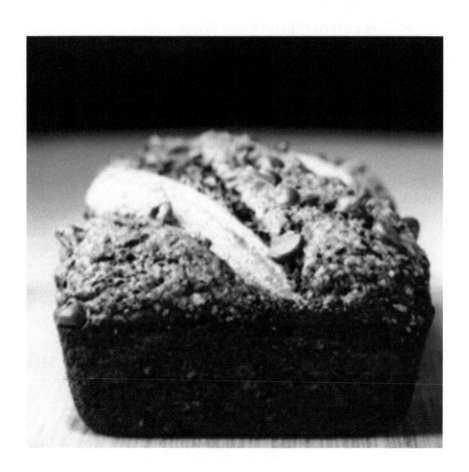

Apple oatmeal bake

Oat is a nutritious ingredient, on the other hand, apple is a healthy fruit that can help to keep the doctor away. As a result, this recipe is a healthy Mediterranean Sea diet rich with fruits and whole foods especially oats.

Ingredients

- ⅔ cup of granulated sugar
- 2 cups of rolled oats
- 2 teaspoons of cinnamon
- 1½ stick of unsalted butter
- 1 cup of walnuts
- 6 large apples

Directions

- In a food processor, process the oats and walnuts until you get flour-like texture.
- Grate the apples with fruit grater.
- In a mixing dish, mix the processed oats together with, walnuts, and sugar.
- Next, oil your ovenproof dish with butter.
- Use the oat mixture to cover the bottom of the oven dish.

- Press down slightly to add half of the apples.

- Cover with more oat mixture on top.

- Repeat this step until everything is done.

- Slice the butter after which cover the whole surface with it.

- Proceed to bake for 35 minutes in a preheated oven at 400°F until golden brown.

- Serve and pour over vanilla pudding if you like.

- Enjoy.

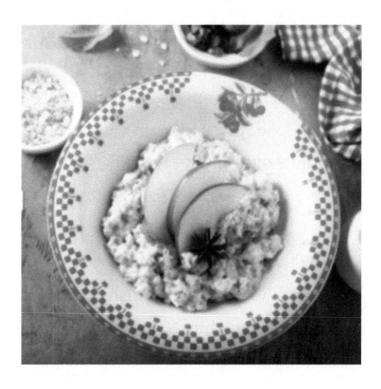

Plum tart with ricotta and Greek yogurt

Ingredients

- 100g of ricotta
- 2 teaspoons of ground cinnamon
- 60g of unsalted butter
- 100g of Greek yogurt
- 2 tablespoons of powdered sugar
- 100g of superfine sugar
- 2 medium eggs
- 2 teaspoons of baking powder
- 160g of all-purpose flour
- 400g of plums

Directions

- Begin by creaming your butter with sugar for about 5 minutes or so.
- Add eggs, one at a time and beat preferably with an electric mixer until fluffy.
- Place in the ricotta into Greek yogurt and mix.
- Then, sift in the flour mixed together with the baking powder and cinnamon.

- Fold in with a wooden spoon to combine all ingredients.
- Cut the plumbs in half after cleaning and remove pits.
- Place onto a baking tray and pour the mixture in the pan, for a silicone cake pan.
- Spread the mixture evenly them top with the plums.
- Proceed to bake for 40 minutes in a preheated oven at 350°F.
- Remove from the oven when ready and let cool totally.
- Dust with some icing sugar.
- Serve and enjoy.

Chocolate Nutella mouse with strawberries

This is a desert with an exciting tasty and sweetness for any occasion. It is easy and quick to make in only 30 minutes, you will be exciting your taste buds with this Mediterranean Sea diet recipe.

Ingredients

- 2 tablespoons of lemon juice
- 2 cups of whipping cream
- 2 tablespoons of caster sugar
- 7 ounces of dark chocolate
- 2 cups of fresh strawberries
- 2 tablespoons of powdered sugar
- 5 tablespoons of Nutella

Directions

- Start by cutting the chocolate into small pieces.
- Over double boiler melt the chocolates with ½ cup of whipping cream. Allow it to cool.

- As the chocolate melts, whip the cream together with the powdered sugar until soft peaks form.
- Then, whisk Nutella with a few tablespoons of whipped cream in a large mixing dish.
- Fold the whipped cream into the Nutella mixture.
- It is time to stir in the cooled chocolate.
- Divide the mousse into 5 glasses or more.
- Place in the refrigerator for 60 minutes.
- As the mousse refrigerates, prepare the strawberries by cleaning, and trimming any green parts.
- Cut into small pieces.
- Shift them into a bowl.
- Add caster sugar and lemon juice.
- Place in a refrigerator 30 minutes.
- Remove and top each glass with strawberries and the juice if any.
- Serve and enjoy.

No bake pineapple cake with Nutella

This incredible desert recipe only features 7 ingredients and gets ready in 20 minutes; a very short time, isn't it? This recipe can be made ahead of time with Nutella and pineapple pieces.

Ingredients

- 1 can of pineapple slices
- 1 ½ cup of sour cream
- 4 tablespoons of Nutella
- 2 tablespoons of powdered sugar
- ½ cup of Greek yogurt
- ½ cup of sour cream
- 3 tablespoons of powdered sugar
- 2 cups of graham crumbs, heaped
- ⅓ cup of unsalted butter

Directions

- Mix melted butter together with the digestive biscuit crumbs. Endeavor to combine well.
- Shift the entire mixture into cake tin, press down to make the crust.

- Drain the pineapple slices of any excess unwanted water and pat them dry.
- Cut 4 – 5 pineapple slices in halves.
- Place them inside the cake pan with others (they should be separate; they should touch each other).
- Any remaining pineapples should be cut into small pieces and spread them over the biscuit layer.
- Whisk together powdered sugar with Nutella and the Sour cream to combined.
- Spread this mixture over the pineapple slices.
- Now, in another separate mixing dish, mix sour cream together with the powdered sugar, and Greek yogurt.
- Spread over Nutella layer.
- Cover this mixture with cling film.
- Move it to the fridge, let refrigerate for at 14 hours.
- You can beautify with pineapples if you like.
- Serve and enjoy.

Strawberry marshmallow brownies

These Mediterranean Sea diet strawberry marshmallow brownies are chewy on the inside. They are delicious and can make a whole breakfast or as a desert.

Ingredients

- 4 Medium Eggs
- 7 ounces of Marshmallows
- 2 cups of Fresh Strawberries
- 7 ounces of Bittersweet
- 3/4 cup of Granulated Sugar
- 2 teaspoon of Baking Powder
- 11/4 cup of All-Purpose Flour
- 1½ stick of Unsalted Butter

Directions

- Melt the chocolate with butter in a pot containing simmering water.
- Allow it to cool when melted.
- Meanwhile, in a large bowl, whisk eggs, then add sugar. Continue to whisk until foamy.
- Adding in flour with the baking powder.
- Mix until smooth.

- Now, add melted chocolate mix to combined.

- Pour this mixture into a large baking pan that is well aligned with baking paper parchment.

- Then, bake for 10 minutes in a preheated oven at 360°F.

- Top with marshmallows together with the strawberries when the 10 minutes have run out.

- Then move it back in the oven in the same pan.

- Continue to bake another 10 minutes.

- Serve and enjoy when ready.

Fried battered apple rings

This is a simple recipe to make in 5 minutes yet delicious and mouth-watering. Here, apple slices are simply dipped into batter, later deep fried and coated with some cinnamon sugar. It is a wonderful Mediterranean recipe to try at home.

Ingredients

- 11/4 cup of vegetable oil
- ½ cup of all-purpose flour
- 3 tablespoons of milk
- 1 teaspoon of ground cinnamon
- 1/4 cup of granulated sugar
- 1 teaspoon of rum
- 2 large apples
- 1 large egg
- 1 tablespoon of granulated sugar

Directions

- Firstly, combine and mix flour together with the milk, rum, egg, sugar until smooth batter in a soup dish.

- Clean and slice apples into thin slices with the core removed.
- Next, heat up oil in a frying pan until shimmering without smoke.
- Get every ring and dip in the batter and fry until all sides turn to golden brown.
- Fry all the 12 apple slices the same way in 5 minutes or so.
- Drain any excess oil with a kitchen towel.
- Coat in cinnamon sugar before they have cooled completely.
- Serve and enjoy.

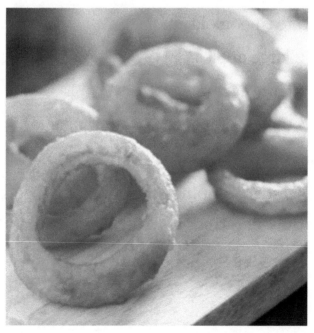

No fuss mixed fruit crisp with hazelnuts

Mediterranean Sea diet emphasizes consumption of vegetable and fruits. Among other several recipes, this no fuss mixed fruit crisp with hazelnuts blends variety of fruits as a tasty desert with fully packed with vitamins.

Ingredients

- 60g of unsalted butter, diced
- 1 kg of mixed fruit mainly apples, peaches, figs
- 20g of unsalted butter
- 100g of plain flour
- 30g of brown sugar
- 2 tablespoons of corn flour
- 50g of hazelnuts , roughly chopped
- 100g of rolled oats
- 40g of brown sugar
- 1 teaspoon of cinnamon

Directions

- Clean the fruits.
- Place all of them into an oven-proof dish.
- Add cinnamon along with hazelnuts, corn flour, and sugar.

- Make sure it is well mixed to spread the ingredients evenly.
- Then, cut the butter into small pieces, place them on top.
- Combine the rolled oats, plain flour, unsalted butter, and brown sugar in a larger bowl.
- Mix thoroughly to combine with your hands.
- Incorporate the butter into the oats mixture.
- Break up the butter blend into the into oats.
- Spread the topping evenly over the fruits.
- Put in a preheated oven to bake for 45 minutes over high heat until the juices just begin to bubble.
- Serve and enjoy with ice cream.

Strawberry banana frozen yogurt

The Mediterranean Sea diet has invented many substitutions to consumption of unhealthy foods. This strawberry banana frozen yogurt is a perfect replacement for ice cream that has high sugar and calorie content.

Ingredients

- 2 tablespoon of honey
- 2 ripe bananas
- Frozen strawberries
- Greek yogurt

Directions

- Firstly, place the strawberries to thaw a bit.
- Then puree in a food processor.
- Place in the peeled and sliced bananas to the mixture.
- Add the yogurt to the mixture continue to process until smooth.
- Taste and adjust accordingly.
- Transfer into a plastic container when tightly covered with a lid.
- Place in freezer and let freeze.

- Remove the container after 2 hours.
- Break the ice with a spoon.
- Serve and enjoy with your required consistency.

No bake banana banoffee pie

This Mediterranean Sea diet is quite flourless and with no eggs as well. the desert only blends bananas as the main flavor to this desert.

Ingredients

- Chocolate
- 1 can of Dulce de Leche
- 10 ounces of Whipping Cream
- 2 Bananas
- ½ cup of Melted butter
- 2 tablespoons Icing Sugar
- 8.8 ounces of Digestive Biscuits

Directions

- Expressly, begin by melting the butter.
- Crush the biscuits into crumbs in a food processor.
- Then, pour over the melted butter let mix until well combined.
- Line the bottom and sides of a round cake tin with baking paper.

- Place two thirds of the biscuit mix in. Make sure to spread the mix evenly.
- Out of the paper, cut a circle and place it over the biscuit crumbs.
- Press down hard enough with your hands to create an even base.
- After this, feel free to discard the baking paper.
- Add biscuit crumbs on the sides of the cake tin, but ensure to create a wall with a spoon.
- Transfer the mixture to refrigerate for 30 minutes.
- As the mixture refrigerates, pour half of the Dulce de Leech into a sauce pan.
- Bring to a boil for 5 minutes, stirring constantly.
- Let it cool little bit.
- Spread it over the chilled biscuit base.
- The remaining half of Dulce de Leche should now be used to spread over the thick layer.
- Cover with the banana slices.
- Pour chilled cream into a chilled dish.
- Now, add icing sugar and whip to make it stiff.

- Spread the cream over the banana layer.
- Place back in the fridge for 1 hour.
- If desired, finish with chocolate shavings.
- Serve and enjoy.

Plum tart with ricotta and Greek yogurt

Ingredients

- 100g of ricotta
- 2 teaspoons of ground cinnamon
- 60g of unsalted butter
- 100g of Greek yogurt
- 2 tablespoons of powdered sugar
- 100g of superfine sugar
- 2 medium eggs
- 2 teaspoons of baking powder
- 160g of all-purpose flour
- 400g of plums

Directions

- Begin by creaming your butter with sugar for about 5 minutes or so.
- Add eggs, one at a time and beat preferably with an electric mixer until fluffy.
- Place in the ricotta into Greek yogurt and mix.
- Then, sift in the flour mixed together with the baking powder and cinnamon.

- Fold in with a wooden spoon to combine all ingredients.
- Cut the plumbs in half after cleaning and remove pits.
- Place onto a baking tray and pour the mixture in the pan, for a silicone cake pan.
- Spread the mixture evenly them top with the plums.
- Proceed to bake for 40 minutes in a preheated oven at 350°F.
- Remove from the oven when ready and let cool totally.
- Dust with some icing sugar.
- Serve and enjoy.

Tahini banana shakes

This banana shakes recipe takes about 5 minutes to make. Interestingly, it can be made ahead of time, but trust me, you will not rest until you have consumed it all at once because of sweetness and irresistible taste.

Ingredients

- 2 sliced frozen bananas
- 4 pitted Medjool dates
- 1/4 cup tahini
- 1/4 cup crushed ice
- 1 ½ cups unsweetened almond milk
- Pinch ground cinnamon

Directions

- Begin by adding the sliced frozen bananas in a blender along with the remaining ingredients at once.
- Keep the blender until a visible smooth and creamy shake.
- Transfer the date shakes to your serving cups.
- Add the pinch ground cinnamon on the top of the cream.

- Enjoy

How to freezing the bananas?

- Slice peeled bananas in to 2 slices.
- Arrange the banana slices in one layer put on a lined sheet pan with parchment paper
- Put in the freezer until the bananas are completely frozen.
- Transfer the frozen bananas to a freezer safe bag and or close tightly in case you want to use at a later time.

The ultimate Mediterranean breakfast

If one is looking for a wholesomely satisfying breakfast, then look not for the answer, it is right here. This breakfast can be packed with falafel, baba ganoush, hummus, and tabbouleh.

Ingredients

- 1 Baba Ganoush Recipe
- Grapes
- Feta cheese
- Extra virgin olive oil and Za'atar to dip
- Pita Bread, sliced into quarters
- 1 Tabbouleh Recipe
- Marinated artichokes or mushrooms
- 1 to 2 tomatoes, sliced
- 1 English cucumber, sliced
- 6 to 7 sliced Radish
- 1 Falafel Recipe
- Assorted olives
- Fresh herbs for garnish
- 1 Classic Hummus Recipe

Directions

- Begin by preparing the falafel recipe at least a night before mainly soaking the chickpeas. Alternatively, one can simply buy the ready falafel.
- Also make the hummus recipe and baba ganoush, a night prior and store in a refrigerator.
- Slice the feta cheese a head of time.
- Make the tabouli in advance. It is okay if it is made days prior but must be kept in tight-lid container and refrigerated.
- To assemble, put the baba ganoush, olive oil, za'atar, hummus, and the tabouli in bowls.
- The largest bowl should be place at the center of a platter for the purposes of creating an easy focal point.
- Place other bowls besides the largest bowl to form shape and easy movement.
- Using the gaps between the bowls, place the remaining ingredients; sliced vegetables, falafel, and pita bread.

- Add the grapes and do not forget to garnish with herbs if desired.
- Serve and enjoy.

Frozen banana pops

Ingredients

- 2 teaspoons chia seeds
- 4 teaspoons freeze dried raspberries
- 4 bananas
- 2 teaspoons pollen
- 2 tablespoons almond butter
- 1 cup Greek yogurt
- 1/4 cup almonds without skin and roughly chopped

Directions

- Cut bananas into halves and place on a tray lined with baking parchment let them freeze for 30 minutes.
- As it freezes, combine the Greek yogurt together with the almond butter and blend well.
- Stick the bananas with an ice pop after you have removed them from the fridge.
- Coat each with yogurt mixture, then place it onto the tray.

- Do this for all the bananas.
- Sprinkle with freeze dried raspberries, chopped almonds, pollen and chia seeds.
- Return the tray back to the freezer to let set for an hour.
- Serve and enjoy when frozen.

Vegan peanut butter banana brownies

If you have never tested a flourless banana brownie, this is your chance to make one for your own. It is gluten free and rich in protein content. Is features dates and banana which are kept fudgy

Ingredients

- 2 cups of pitted dates
- 1/4 cup of coconut oil , melted
- 2 tablespoon of water
- ⅓ cup of unsweetened cocoa powder
- ⅓ cup of peanut butter
- 1 large banana, ripe
- A pinch of salt

Directions

- Preheat your oven to 356°F
- Place the dates, coconut oil, and water in a food processor.
- Process until it forms a paste.
- Add cocoa powder, banana, peanut butter, and salt after it has formed the paste.
- Process until smooth.

- Shift the entire mixture into a pan lined with baking parchment.
- Then, bake for 10 minutes.
- Let cool when ready.
- Slice and enjoy.

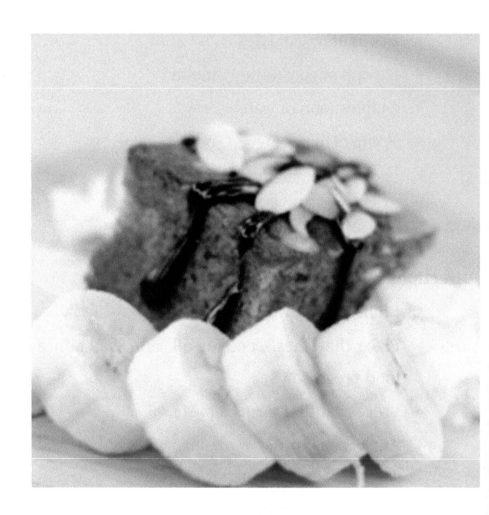

Spiced cocoa roasted almonds

This is mainly a snack recipe. They are very delicious especially when covered with cocoa.

Ingredients

- 2 tablespoons of brown sugar
- 1 tablespoon of water
- ½ cup of brown sugar
- 1 teaspoon of ground cinnamon
- 1/4 teaspoon of ground cinnamon
- 7 ounces of almonds , raw
- ½ teaspoon of ground nutmeg
- 1 tablespoon of unsweetened cocoa powder
- 1/4 teaspoon of cardamom
- ½ teaspoon of sea salt
- 1/4 teaspoon of anise
- 1 egg white

Directions

- Combine the egg white with water and whisk until frothy.
- Add sugar together with the spices and salt mix thoroughly.

- Place in the almonds blend well to coat.
- Transfer the mixture to a baking tray aligned with baking parchment.
- Spread the mixture around in one layer.
- Bake in a preheated oven at 300°F for 30 minutes.
- Endeavor to stir as it bakes gently.
- Shift the roasted almonds into a sauce pan with cocoa, sugar, cinnamon.
- Shake the mixture with the lid closed to coat the almond.
- Let cool.
- Serving and enjoy.

Double chocolate oatmeal

Chocolate oatmeal is a recipe with rich carbohydrate content and fiber making it a perfect Mediterranean Sea diet choice for an energy giving breakfast. It is chocolate flavored sweetened with honey or syrup topping with strawberries.

Ingredients

- 1/4 cup of chocolate chips
- 12 fresh strawberries
- 1 cup of water
- A pinch of salt
- 1 cup of milk
- 4 tablespoons of maple syrup
- 1 cup of rolled oats
- 2 tablespoon of unsweetened cocoa powder

Directions

- Roll the oats, together milk, salt and water in a pot.
- Bring to a boil when covered.
- Lower the heat and open the lid.

- Add cocoa powder and stir frequently for 7minutes.
- Stir in the maple syrup and chocolate chips when the heat is turned off.
- Place in 2 serving dishes.
- Serve when topped with strawberries and chocolate chips.
- Enjoy.

Quinoa egg muffins

Eggs are known for the provision of most food nutrients. They are juicy and very flavorful for a delicious breakfast.

Ingredients

- a pinch of black pepper
- 1 large carrot, grated
- ½ tsp salt
- ½ leek, chopped
- 1 green pepper, diced
- 3 ounce of cheddar cheese, grated
- 2 tablespoons of Greek yogurt
- ½ zucchini
- 2 tablespoons of dried oregano
- 2 tablespoons of extra virgin olive oil
- ½ cup of uncooked quinoa
- 2 eggs, small-medium

Directions

- Preheat your oven at 350°F.
- Start by cooking quinoa as per the manufacturers package Directions.
- Let cool briefly.

- Heat olive oil in the frying pan.
- Add chopped leek, diced pepper, grated carrot, and diced zucchini let Sauté for 10 minutes.
- Stir in the oregano.
- Season with salt accordingly.
- In a bowl, beat the eggs mixing with the yogurt, and salt.
- Add black pepper, grated cheese, and cooled quinoa.
- Add sautéed veggies mix thoroughly to blend and combine.
- Align a muffin tray with paper
- Place the mixture in all the spots in the tray.
- Bake in the preheated oven for 20 minutes.
- Serve and enjoy.

Sweet potato burgers

Sweet potato burger is a whole meal Mediterranean Sea diet vegetable burger made with buckwheat.

Ingredients

- Guacamole
- ½ cup of buckwheat
- 1 tablespoon of <u>curry powder</u>
- 2 large tomatoes
- 1 small onion
- 2 carrots
- ½ cucumber
- 3 cups of diced sweet potatoes
- 2 tablespoons of <u>extra virgin olive oil</u>
- 1/4 red cabbage
- Salt and pepper to taste
- ½ cup of packed fresh parsley
- 6 buns

Directions

- Place the sweet potatoes in a sauce pan.
- Add in water to cover them all.
- Boil covered with lid.

- After it has boiled for 6 minutes, lower the heat and continue to cook until soft in 4 minutes or so.
- Drain any excess water and set aside.
- As the potatoes are cooking, cook the buckwheat following the package Directions.
- Sauté onions and carrots in a skillet with some olive oil until onions are translucent.
- Shift the potatoes into a mixing bowl.
- Using a potato masher, mash them with a fork.
- Introduce the remaining ingredients and mix well.
- Use part of the mixture and roll it into a ball.
- Move it onto a baking tray.
- Make sure the tray is aligned with parchment paper.
- Repeat this for all the mixture.
- Bake in already heated oven at 360°F for 10 minutes.
- Turn the other side, continue to bake for another 10 minutes.
- Serve with buns and lots of veggies.

- Enjoy.

Blueberry coffee breakfast smoothie

The exciting flavor of coffee takes control of this smoothie. It features blueberry with natural sweetness for a healthy and tasty breakfast.

Ingredients

- 6 dates , pitted
- ½ cup of rolled oats
- 2 teaspoons of instant coffee
- 1 cup of almond milk
- 1 cup of fresh blueberries

Directions

- In a blender, combine the oats together with the blueberries, dates, instant coffee, and milk.
- Bland until finely smooth.
- Serve and enjoy immediately.

Apricot coconut popsicles

Apricot coconut popsicles are frozen treat with a refreshing healthy taste and so easy and quick to make in 10 minutes.

Ingredients

- 3 tablespoons of coconut oil
- 3 tablespoons of honey
- 1/4 cup of coconut milk
- 2 cups of apricots, pitted and halved

Directions

- Place all ingredients in a food processor, process until smooth.
- Pour the mixture into the popsicle molds with inserted sticks.
- Freeze for not less than 4 hours.
- Serve and enjoy.

793. Cherry avocado chocolate mousse

This is a perfect healthy desert with no added artificial sugar. These cherry avocado chocolate mousse features a rich chocolate flavor, creamy avocado and cherries and dates from where it derives its sweetness.

Ingredients

- ⅛ teaspoon of pink salt
- ½ cup of coconut milk drink
- 1 cup of cherries, stoned
- ½ cup of dates
- 2 large avocados
- ½ cup of natural unsweetened cocoa powder

Directions

- Start by soaking the dates in water for 30 minutes.
- Cut avocados in half.
- Using a spoon, scoop out the flesh, put in a food processor.
- Add cocoa powder together with the dates, coconut milk drink, cherries, and salt.
- Process until smooth and creamy.
- Use the cherries to beautify.
- Serve and enjoy.

Ricotta chocolate banana toast with seeds

This breakfast can keep you until your next meal time. It is basically a whole wheat toast in 10 minutes.

Ingredients

- 2 teaspoons of honey
- 1 cup ricotta
- 4 slices of toast bread
- 4 teaspoons of mixed seed
- 2 large bananas
- 2 ounces of dark chocolate

Directions

- Begin by toasting your bread using a toaster.
- Combine ricotta with honey as the bread toasts.
- Taste and adjust accordingly.
- Melt the chocolate over a pot of simmering water.
- Spread it over every toasted bread.
- Add ricotta mixture with the sliced banana and seeds.
- If you like, garnish with grated chocolate.

- Serve and enjoy.

Homemade strawberry jam with brown sugar

The uniqueness with this recipe is that it has no artificial preservatives making it a health Mediterranean diet for a breakfast.

Ingredients

- 2.2 pounds of strawberries
- 1½ lemon
- ½ pound of brown sugar

Directions

- Hull the strawberries and cut into small pieces.
- Refrigerate in a bowl.
- Place in a large pot. Stir with vigor for 5 minutes over medium heat.
- Make sure they turn mushy.
- Add sugar together with the lemon juice.
- Cook for 35 minutes or until the jam is thick while stirring frequently.
- It is time to remove the saucer from the fridge.
- Spread with some jam.

- Let it cool down and check its thickness by drawing a line through.
- Cook it further, if the jam does not fill the space of the drawn line.
- Otherwise, pour into sterilized jugs leaving 1 cm free from the top.
- Seal properly, then turn up-side down.
- Let it settle for at least 30 minutes.
- Return the jugs to an upright position.
- Serve and enjoy.

Blueberry turnovers

The recipe combines puff pastry together with homemade blueberry fillings. This Mediterranean diet is fit for breakfast, lunch or dinner.

Ingredients

- All-purpose flour , for dusting
- ⅓ cup brown sugar
- 1 tablespoon lemon juice
- 1 teaspoon brown sugar
- 1 small egg, beaten
- 2 ounces unsalted butter
- 2 teaspoons cornstarch
- 1 sheet puff pastry, thawed or fresh
- 2 cups frozen blueberries

Directions

- Combine blueberries, sugar with the lemon juice and simmer for 10 minutes in a small saucepan.
- Follow by stirring in the butter.
- Make sure to dilute cornstarch in 1 tablespoon of water in a cup.

- Add bit of the blueberry sauce, stir well to mix.
- Pour the cornstarch into the saucepan, make sure to stir until the sauce is thick.
- Pour it into a bowl when ready, let cool for 30 minutes.
- Preheat an oven to 400°F.
- Unfold the puff pastry and roll it out.
- Cut into squares.
- Scoop 2 heaped teaspoons blueberry filling in the middle of pastry squares.
- Run your finger alongside the sides of each square after dipping your finger in water.
- Lift one tip of the pastry and fold it over the filling towards the opposite tip forming a triangle.
- To seal, press down the edges.
- Double-seal with a fork.
- Place turnovers onto a baking tray.
- Pierce each turnover to allow steam to escape.
- Brush with egg wash and sprinkle with brown sugar.
- Bake in the oven for 15 minutes.

- When ready, serve and enjoy.

Strawberry coconut tart

This recipe uses simple and easy to find ingredients. It is quite easy to make from scratch in 35 minutes.

Ingredients

- 2/3 cups of unsweetened desiccated coconut
- 1 stick unsalted butter , melted
- 4 tablespoons of strawberry jam
- 3 tablespoons of powdered sugar
- 1 cup of all-purpose flour
- ½ cup of powdered sugar
- 1 egg white, from a large egg

Directions

- In a mixing bowl, combine flour with powdered sugar.
- Add melted butter.
- Make sure to mix thoroughly with a large spoon.
- Mix your hands when it begins to form dough.
- Wrap it and let chill for 30 minutes.
- Remove it from the fridge and fill the bottom and sides of a pie pan with it. Do not roll.

- Take a piece of the pastry and press it down. This should be piece by piece until you use up all of it.
- Spread jam over the crust. Keep aside.
- Whip the egg white until soft peaks appear.
- Add sifted sugar and beat until smooth.
- Stir in the coconut.
- Pour this mixture over the jam and spread evenly round.
- Bake in a preheated oven at 350°F for 25-30 minutes.
- Remove out when ready and let it cool totally.
- Serve and enjoy.

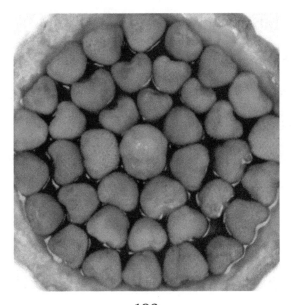

Mango panna cotta

Though a perfect Mediterranean Sea diet, mango panna cotta an Italian desert wonderful picnics, parties and dinners. It can be prepared ahead of time.

Ingredients

- A knob of butter
- ½ cup of whole milk
- ½ teaspoon of vanilla essence
- 1 cup of heavy cream the whole package
- 1 packet gelatin
- ½ lemon, juice only
- 2 cups of frozen mango chunks, thawed
- ⅓ cup of granulated sugar
- 2 tablespoons of granulated sugar

Directions

- Pour heavy cream together with the milk and sugar into a small sauce pan.
- Stir to dissolve the sugar on over low heat, the cream should be hot.
- Turn off the heat and stir vanilla essence. Make sure not to boil at this stage.

- The bloom should be gelatin as per the package Directions.
- Add the bloomed gelatin to the cooled cream mixture. Do not forget to mix to dissolve.
- Pour the mixture into small glasses, place to refrigerate to set the panna cotta for 2 hours.
- Process the thawed mango pieces together with the lemon juice and sugar in a blender until smooth.
- Taste and adjust accordingly.
- Simmer in a small saucepan over low heat.
- Stir in butter to get a much creamier texture.
- Allow the mixture to cool.
- Pour over the panna cotta.
- Serve and enjoy.

Candied oranges dipped in chocolate

This recipe is for a sweet tasty treat for a perfect holiday to enjoy Mediterranean Sea diet. The chocolates can be substituted with cupcakes if you like.

Ingredients

- 3.5 ounces of Dark Chocolate
- 1 Large Orange, organic
- Coarse Salt
- 1 cup of Granulated Sugar
- 1 cup of Water

Directions

- Cut the oranges into thin slices.
- Heat water and sugar in a large pot until the sugar has dissolved.
- Add the orange slices in a manner that they are spread around without covering each other totally.
- Let simmer for 40 minutes on a low heat. Turn occasionally.
- Transfer slices onto a wire rack when ready, let them cool completely.

- It is fine to cool on a fridge to speed up the cooling process.
- Melt the chocolate over a pot of simmering water.
- Dip half of each slice in chocolate.
- Place the dipped one's onto a tray lined with a sheet of aluminum foil.
- Sprinkle with salt.
- Shift all of them into the fridge.
- Serve an enjoy.

Walnut crescent cookies

If you want taste and know divine taste covered in a powdered sugar, look no further, walnut crescent cookies can give you that same exact taste.

Ingredients

- 2 tablespoons of vanilla sugar
- 11/4 cup of all-purpose flour
- ½ cup of powdered sugar
- 1 stick unsalted butter
- ⅔ cup of ground walnuts
- 4 tablespoons of powdered sugar
- 1 teaspoon of vanilla essence

Directions

- In a large mixing bowl, begin by combining sifted powdered sugar, sifted flour, and ground walnuts.
- Next, add vanilla essence and mix thoroughly.
- Then, grate chilled butter.
- Add to the bowl.

- Combine all the ingredients using your bare hands until dough is formed in 3 minutes or so.
- Place into a Ziploc bag allow it to chill for 30 minutes in the fridge.
- As it refrigerates, get a small bowl and place extra powdered sugar with vanilla sugar in it and keep aside.
- Take a piece of the dough and roll into a ball then into a sausage.
- Shape the sausage into a crescent.
- Place onto a baking tray with baking parchment.
- For the remaining dough, repeat this step.
- Bake in a ready heated oven at 400°F for 8 minutes or so.
- Allow it to cool down completely on the tray when already fried.
- Transfer to a plat and dip with powdered sugar to coat.
- Serve and enjoy.

Lightning Source UK Ltd.
Milton Keynes UK
UKHW020635280521
384530UK00001B/54

9 781802 696332